KETO DIET

A Little Cookbook To Start Your Transformation Today – Lose Weight In 21 Days

Adele Glenn

.

Table of Contents

Introduction

For the benefits of weight loss, the ketogenic diet has been widely commended and praised. It has been shown that this high-fat, low-carb diet is highly balanced overall. It really makes your body, like a talking machine, burn fat. It is also respected by public figures. But the question is, how can ketosis increase the loss of weight? The following is a comprehensive picture of the process of ketosis and weight loss.

Ketosis is considered rare by some people. Even though several nutritionists and physicians have approved it. It is still disapproved of by many people. The misconceptions are attributable to the myths about the ketogenic diet that have spread.

When the body is out of glucose, it relies on stored fat immediately. It is also important to note that glucose is created by carbohydrates and you will also be able to lower your glucose levels once you begin a low carbohydrate diet. Then, instead of carbohydrates, that is, glucose, your body can generate fuel by fat.

The mechanism of accumulating fat via fat is known as ketosis, and it becomes extremely effective at burning excess fat once your body enters this state. Also, as during the ketogenic diet, glucose levels are low, the body gains many other health benefits.

A ketogenic diet is not only good for weight loss, it also helps in a positive way to boost your overall health. Ketogenic focuses on placing the body in a natural metabolic state, that is, ketosis, unlike all other diet plans, which focus on decreasing calorie intake. The only thing that makes this diet controversial is that it is not very well thought out for this kind of metabolism. Your body will easily burn accumulated fat by having tattoos on your body regularly, leading to great weight loss.

The query arises now. How does the human body become affected by ketosis? This process does not last more than 2-3 days, however. This is the time the human body takes to reach the process of ketosis. You are not going to have any side effects until you get in.

You should also begin reducing the consumption of calories and carbohydrates gradually. The most common mistake dietitians make is that, at the same time, they want to begin removing something from their diet. This is where the issue occurs. When you restrict all at once, the human body can respond extremely negatively. You've got to begin gradually. Read this guide to learn more about how the ketogenic diet can be treated after 50.

Most fats are healthy and important to our health, so essential fatty acids and essential amino acids are available (proteins). The most powerful source of energy is fat, and every gram contains around 9 calories. This more than doubles the sum of protein and carbohydrates (both have 4 calories per gram).

Your body adjusts and converts the fat and protein, as well as the fat it has accumulated, into ketones or ketones for energy when you consume a lot of fat and protein and substantially reduce carbohydrates. This mechanism of metabolism is called ketosis. The ketogen in the ketogenic diet comes from here.

CHAPTER 1:

Breakfast

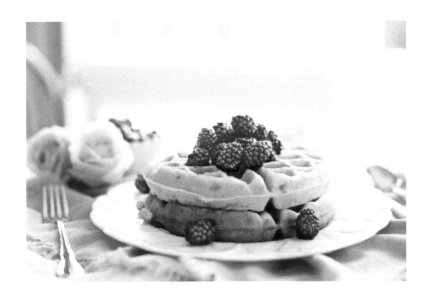

1. Capicola Egg Cups

Preparation Time: 5 minutes

Cooking Time: 15 minutes

Servings: 4

Ingredients:

- 8 eggs
- 1 cup cheddar cheese
- 4 oz. capicola or bacon (slices)
- salt, pepper, basil

Directions:

1. Preheat the oven to 400°F. You will need 8 wells of a standard-size muffin pan.
2. Place the slices in the 8 wells, forming a cup shape. Sprinkle into each cup some of the cheese, according to your liking.
3. Crack an egg into each cup, season them with salt and pepper.
4. Bake for 10-15 mins. Serve hot, top it with basil.

Nutrition:

Carbs: 1 g

Fat: 11 g

Protein: 16 g

Calories: 171 kcal

2.   Overnight "noats"

Preparation Time: 5 minutes plus overnight to chill

Cooking Time: 10 minutes

Servings: 1

Ingredients:

- 2 tablespoons hulled hemp seeds
- 1 tablespoon chia seeds
- ½ scoop (about 8 grams) collagen powder
- ½ cup unsweetened nut or seed milk (hemp, almond, coconut, and cashew)

Direction:

1. In a small mason jar or glass container, combine the hemp seeds, chia seeds, collagen, and milk.
2. Secure tightly with a lid, shake well, and refrigerate overnight.

Nutrition:

Calories: 263

 Total Fat: 19g

Protein: 16g

Total Carbs: 7g

Fiber: 5g

Net Carbs: 2g

3.   Frozen keto coffee

Preparation Time: 5 minutes

Cooking Time: 20 minutes

Servings: 1

Ingredients:

- 12 ounces coffee, chilled
- 1 scoop MCT powder (or 1 tablespoon MCT oil)
- 1 tablespoon heavy (whipping) cream
- Pinch ground cinnamon
- Dash sweetener (optional)
- ½ cup ice

Directions:

1. In a blender, combine the coffee, MCT powder, cream, cinnamon, sweetener (if using), and ice. Blend until smooth.

Nutrition:

Calories: 127;

Total Fat: 13g;

Protein: 1g;

Total Carbs: 1.5g;

Fiber: 1g;

Net Carbs: 0.5g

4.   Easy Skillet Pancakes

Preparation Time: 5 minutes

Cooking Time: 5 minutes

Servings: 8

Ingredients:

- 8 ounces cream cheese
- 8 eggs
- 2 tablespoons coconut flour
- 2 teaspoons baking powder
- 1 teaspoon ground cinnamon
- ½ teaspoon vanilla extract
- 1 teaspoon liquid stevia or sweetener of choice (optional)
- 2 tablespoons butter

Directions

1. In a blender, combine the cream cheese, eggs, coconut flour, baking powder, cinnamon, vanilla, and stevia (if using). Blend until smooth.
2. In a large skillet over medium heat, melt the butter.
3. Use half the mixture to pour four evenly sized pancakes and cook for about a minute, until you see bubbles on top. Flip the pancakes and cook for another minute. Remove from the pan and add more butter or oil to the skillet if needed. Repeat with the remaining batter.

4. Top with butter and eat right away, or freeze the pancakes in a freezer-safe resealable bag with sheets of parchment in between, for up to 1 month.

Nutrition:

Calories: 179

Total Fat: 15g

Protein: 8g

Total Carbs: 3g

Fiber: 1g

Net Carbs: 2g

CHAPTER 2:

Lunch

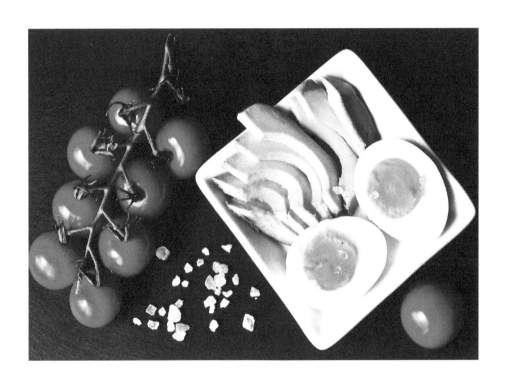

5.   Cheesy Chicken Cauliflower

Preparation Time: 5 minutes

Cooking Time: 10 minutes

Servings: 4

Ingredients:

- 2 cups cauliflower florets, chopped
- ½ cup red bell pepper, chopped
- 1 cup roasted chicken, shredded (Lunch Recipes: Roasted Lemon Chicken Sandwich)
- ¼ cup shredded cheddar cheese
- 1 tablespoon. butter
- 1 tablespoon. sour cream
- Salt and pepper to taste

Directions:

1. Stir fry the cauliflower and peppers in the butter over medium heat until the veggies are tender.
2. Add the chicken and cook until the chicken is warmed through.
3. Add the remaining ingredients and stir until the cheese is melted.
4. Serve warm.

Nutrition:

Calories: 144 kcal

Carbs: 4 g

Fat: 8.5 g

Protein: 13.2 g.

6. Chicken Avocado Salad

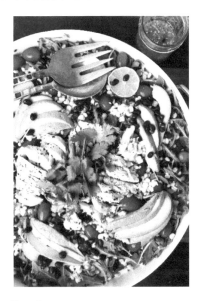

Preparation Time: 7 minutes

Cooking Time: 10 minutes

Servings: 4

Ingredients:

- 1 cup roasted chicken, shredded (Lunch Recipes: Roasted Lemon Chicken Sandwich)
- 1 bacon strip, cooked and chopped
- 1/2 medium avocado, chopped
- ¼ cup cheddar cheese, grated
- 1 hard-boiled egg, chopped
- 1 cup romaine lettuce, chopped
- 1 tablespoon. olive oil
- 1 tablespoon. apple cider vinegar

- Salt and pepper to taste

Directions:

1. Create the dressing by mixing apple cider vinegar, oil, salt and pepper.
2. Combine all the other ingredients in a mixing bowl.
3. Drizzle with the dressing and toss.
4. Can be refrigerated for up to 3 days.

Nutrition:

Calories: 220 kcal

Carbs: 2.8 g

Fat: 16.7 g

Protein: 14.8 g.

7.   Chicken Broccoli Dinner

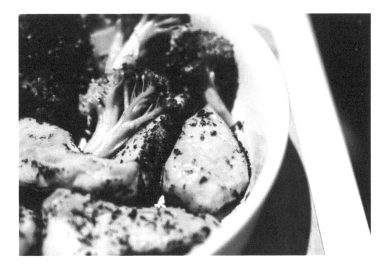

Preparation Time: 10 minutes

Cooking Time: 5 minutes

Servings: 1

Ingredients:

- 1 roasted chicken leg (Lunch Recipes: Roasted Lemon Chicken Sandwich)
- ½ cup broccoli florets
- ½ tablespoon. unsalted butter, softened
- 2 garlic cloves, minced
- Salt and pepper to taste

Directions:

1. Boil the broccoli in lightly salted water for 5 minutes. Drain the water from the pot and keep the broccoli in the pot. Keep the lid on to keep the broccoli warm.

2. Mix all the butter, garlic, salt and pepper in a small bowl to create garlic butter.

3. Place the chicken, broccoli and garlic butter.

Nutrition:

Calories: 257 kcal

Carbs: 5.1 g

Fat: 14 g

Protein: 27.4 g.

CHAPTER 3:

Dinner Recipes

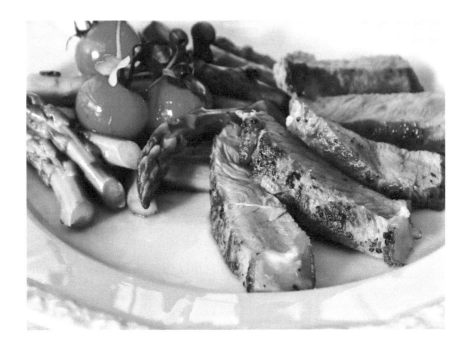

8. Keto Gingerbread Crème Brule

Preparation Time: 15 minutes

Cooking Time: 30 minutes

Servings: 6

Ingredients:

- 1¾ cups heavy whipping cream
- 2 tsp pumpkin pie spice
- 2 tbsperythritol (an all-natural sweetener)
- ¼ tsp vanilla extract
- 4 egg yolks
- ½ clementine (optional)

Directions:

1. Preheat the oven to 360°F.
2. Crack the eggs to separate them and place the egg whites and the egg yolks in two separate bowls. We will only use egg yolks in this recipe, so save the egg whites for a rainy day.
3. Add some cream to a saucepan and bring it to a boil along with the spices, vanilla extract, and sweetener mixed in.
4. Add the warm cream mixture into the egg yolks. Do this slowly, only adding a little bit at a time, while whisking.
5. Pour it into oven-proof ramekins or small Pyrex bowls that are firmly placed in a larger baking dish with large sides.
6. Add some water to the larger dish with the ramekins in it until it's about halfway up the ramekins. Make sure not to get water

in the ramekins though. The water helps the cream cook gently and evenly for a creamy and smooth result.

7. Bake it in the oven for about 30 minutes. Take the ramekins out from the baking dish and let the dessert cool.

8. You can enjoy this dessert either warm or cold, you can also add a clementine segment on top of it.

Nutrition:

Calories: 321

Protein: 14 Grams

Fat: 1 Grams

Net Carbs: 11 Gram

9.   Tuscan Chicken

Preparation Time: 10 minutes

Cooking Time: 30 minutes

Servings: 2

Ingredients:

- 1 lb. boneless and skinless chicken thighs
- 3 tbsps. olive oil
- 6 green onions, chopped
- 1 1/2 cups white wine
- 1 1/2 cups chicken broth
- 1 branch of fresh rosemary
- 1/3 cup black and green olives, pitted and roughly chopped
- Salt and pepper

Directions:

1. In a large skillet, brown the chicken in the oil. Salt lightly (be careful, the olives are already salted) and pepper.
2. Add green onions and continue cooking for about 2 minutes. Add half of the white wine and simmer until evaporated.
3. Add half of the broth, rosemary, and olives. Simmer on low heat until the liquid has reduced by half.
4. Add the remaining wine and broth gradually during cooking as soon as the liquid has reduced by half (see note). Return the chicken a few times during cooking to coat it well in the sauce.

5. Simmer over low heat for about 30 minutes, until the chicken becomes fluffy; check that with a fork and check if the sauce has thickened.

6. Adjust seasoning. Remove the rosemary branch.

7. Divide the chicken thighs between 2 containers

8. Lock the containers and store your dinner in the refrigerator

9. Storage, freeze, thaw and reheat guideline:

10. This Tuscan Chicken can be stored in the refrigerator at 40 °F in a plastic container for about 2 days. When you want to consume your dinner, remove the chicken from the refrigerator and microwave it for about 5 minutes.

Nutrition:

Calories: 505

Fat: 42 g

Carbs: 5.8 g

Protein 26 g

Sugar: 1 g;

10.   Steak with Broccoli

Preparation Time: 5 minutes

Cooking Time: 5 minutes

Servings: 3

Ingredients:

- 1/2 small thinly sliced red onion
- 3 tbsp of red wine vinegar
- 1 pinch of kosher salt
- 1 Pinch of freshly ground black pepper
- 5 tbsp of divided extra-virgin olive oil
- 1 and 1/4 lb. of cut skirt steak
- 1 tsp of ground coriander
- 1 thinly sliced small head of broccoli
- 4 c. of Mache
- 1/4 Cup roasted sunflower seeds
- 4 oz., 1/4 cup shaved ricotta

Directions:

1. Combine the vinegar and about 1/2 tsp. salt in a bowl. Then set it aside

2. Meanwhile, press the function sauté of your Instant pot and heat about 1 tbsp. in it; then season the steak with the coriander, the salt, and the pepper.

3. Lock the lid of your Instant Pot

4. Cook for about 5 minutes at a temperature of 365°F

5. Add the broccoli, the Mache, the sunflower seeds, and the remaining 4 tbsps. oil to the onions and toss to combine it.

6. Season the steak with 1 pinch of salt and the pepper.

7. Storage, freeze, thaw and reheat guideline:

8. To store your dinner, divide it between 3 containers; then put the containers in the refrigerator at a temperature of about 40°F. When you are ready to serve your dinner, remove the containers from the refrigerator and microwave it for about 4 minutes

Nutrition:

Calories: 460

Fat: 37.6g

Carbs: 8.5 g

Protein 21.7g

Sugar: 2.3g

11.   Instant Pot Ketogenic Chili

Preparation Time: 5 minutes

Cooking Time: 30 minutes

Servings: 2

Ingredients:

- 1 lb. of ground Beef
- 1 lb. of ground Sausage
- 1 Medium, chopped green Bell Pepper
- 1/2 Medium, chopped yellow onion
- 1 can of 6 oz. of tomato paste
- 2 tbsps. olive oil
- 1 tbsp. avocado oil
- 1 Tbsp of chili Powder
- ½ Tbsp of ground Cumin
- 3 to 4 minced garlic cloves
- 1/3 to ½ cup water
- 1 can of 14.05 diced tomatoes in the tomato Juice

Directions:

1. Preheat your Instant pot by pressing the "Sauté" button
2. Add in the olive oil and avocado oil; then add the ground beef and the sausage to the Instant pot and cook until it becomes brown.
3. Once the meat is browned set the Instant Pot to the function "keep warm/cancel."

4. Add in the rest of the **Ingredients:** into your Instant Pot and mix very well.

5. Cover the lid of the instant pot and lock it; then make sure that the steam valve is sealed

6. Select the function Bean/Chilli setting for around 30 minutes

7. Once the chili is perfectly cooked, the Instant Pot will automatically shift to the function mode "Keep Warm

8. Let the pressure release naturally, or you can rather use the quick release method.

9. Divide the chili between 2 containers; then top with chopped parsley

10. Store the containers in the refrigerator for two days

Nutrition:

Calories: 555

Fat: 46.5g

Carbs: 9.1 g

Protein 24.9g

Sugar: 3g

12. Ahi Tuna Bowl

Preparation Time: 10 minutes

Cooking Time: 5 minutes

Servings: 2

Ingredients:

- 1 lb. of diced ahi tuna, chopped
- 1 tbsp of coconut Aminos
- ½ tsp of sesame oil
- 1/4 cup mayonnaise
- 2 tbsps. cream cheese
- 2 Tbsps. sriracha
- 1 Diced, ripe avocado
- 1/2 cup Kimchi
- ½ Cup chopped green onion
- 1 tbsp. avocado oil
- 1 pinch of sesame seeds

Directions:

1. Add the avocado oil to the bowl; then add the diced tuna.
2. Add the coconut aminos, the cream cheese, the sesame oil, the mayo, the sriracha to the bowl and toss it very well to combine.
3. Add the diced avocado and the kimchi to the bowl and combine it very well.

4. Divide the Kimchi between two containers; then add the greens, the cauliflower rice and the chopped green onion with the sesame seeds

5. Store the containers in the refrigerator for 2 days.

Nutrition:

Calories: 345

Fat: 26.5 g

Carbs: 6.6 g

Protein 19.8 g

Sugar: 1.4g

13.　Stuffed Spinach and Beef Burgers

Preparation Time: 5 minutes

Cooking Time: 8 minutes

Servings: 2

Ingredients:

- 1 lb. of ground chuck roast
- 1 tsp. salt
- ¾ tsp. ground black pepper
- 2 tbsps. cream cheese
- 1 tbsp. avocado oil
- 1 cup firmly packed fresh spinach
- ½ cup shredded mozzarella cheese (4 to 5 oz.)
- 2 tbsps. grated Parmesan cheese

Directions:

1. In a large bowl, combine the ground beef with the salt, and the pepper.
2. Scoop about 1/3 cup the mixture and with wet hands; shape about 4 patties about ½-inch of thickness. Place the patties in the refrigerator.
3. Place the spinach in a saucepan over medium-high heat.
4. Cover the pan and cook for about 2 minutes, until the spinach becomes wilted.
5. Drain the spinach and let cool; then squeeze the spinach
6. Cut the spinach and put it in a bowl; then stir in the mozzarella cheese, the cream cheese, the avocado oil, and the Parmesan.

7. Scoop ¼ cup the stuffing and shape 4 patties; then cover with the remaining 4 patties

8. Seal both the edges of each burger

9. Cup each of the patties with your hands to make it round

10. Press each of the patties a little bit to make a thick layer Heat your grilling pan over a high heat

11. Grill your burgers for about 6 minutes on each of the two sides.

12. Divide the burgers between 2 containers

13. Store in the refrigerator Serve!

Nutrition:

Calories: 450

Fat: 37 g

Carbs: 7 g

Protein 22 g

Sugar: 1.9g

14.   Ketogenic Low Carb Cloud Bread

Preparation Time: 10 minutes **Cooking Time:** 15 minutes

Servings: 3

Ingredients:

- 1 tsp. baking powder
- 1 Cup Philadelphia cheese
- 3 Organic egg

Directions:

1. Separate the whites from the yolks of the three eggs. Place the whites in one bowl and the yolks in the other.
2. Add the cheese at room temperature to the yolks and mix with an electric mixer to obtain a fine paste.
3. Add the baking soda to the egg whites and mix with the mixer. Mix both mixtures gently with a spatula.
4. Preheat the oven to 300°F. Spread small circles of dough on parchment paper
5. , cook for 15 to 20 minutes.
6. Once the cloud bread is cooked, set it aside to cool for about 5 minutes
7. Divide the cloud bread between 3 plastic wraps; then plastic the plastic wraps in two containers Store the containers in the refrigerator for 3 days

Nutrition:

Calories: 200 Fat: 17g Carbs: 2 g Protein 10g

Sugar: 3g

15. Ketogenic Bruschetta

Preparation Time: 10 minutes

Cooking Time: 45 minutes

Servings: 3

Ingredients:

- 1 tsp. baking powder
- 1 Cup Philadelphia cheese
- 3 Organic egg
- 1 and ½ cups black olives
- 1 caper
- 24 cherry tomatoes
- oregano
- olive oil
- 1 clove of garlic

Directions:

1. Wash, dry and put the peppers on a baking sheet covered with parchment paper.
2. Bake at 400° F for one hour, turning over on the other side after 30 minutes.
3. Put the roasted peppers in a food bag for 15 minutes.
4. Clean the peppers removing the skin and seeds.
5. Put the peppers on a plate and season with olive oil
6. Wash, dry and halve the cherry tomatoes.
7. Heat a peel and roast the tomatoes on both sides.

8. Toss the slices of Pan Bruschetta so that they are crunchy on the outside.

9. Rub the clove of garlic on the slices of bread.

10. Put the pitted olives in the bowl of a blender and mash them.

11. Coat the slices with olive puree, then cover with peppers cut in fillets, add the tomatoes, some capers, sprinkle with oregano and drizzle with a little olive oil

Nutrition:

Calories: 410

Fat: 35g

Carbs: 7.5 g

Protein 16g

Sugar: 1g

16.   Cauliflower Pizza

Preparation Time: 10 minutes

Cooking Time: 20 minutes

Servings: 2

Ingredients:

- 1 cauliflower
- ½ cup grated mozzarella
- 1 organic egg
- 1 cup white ham
- 1 cup mozzarella
- 4 tbsp of tomato sauce
- ½ cup grated cheese
- 1 tsp. oregano

Directions:

1. Cut the cauliflower head into small florets
2. Grate the cauliflower; the heat it for 4 minutes in the microwave
3. Fluff the cauliflower with a fork
4. Mix the egg and grated cheese with drained cauliflower until you obtain the dough
5. Spread the obtained mixture on a sheet of parchment paper and bake at 400°F until golden brown for about 15 to 20 minutes.
6. Garnish your pizza with olive and capers and
7. It's ready

8. Cut the pizza; then divide the portions between 2 containers and store it in the refrigerator for 2 days

Nutrition:

Calories: 430

Fat: 35.4g

Carbs: 7 g

Protein 22.8g

Sugar: 3g

CHAPTER 4:

Soup and Stew

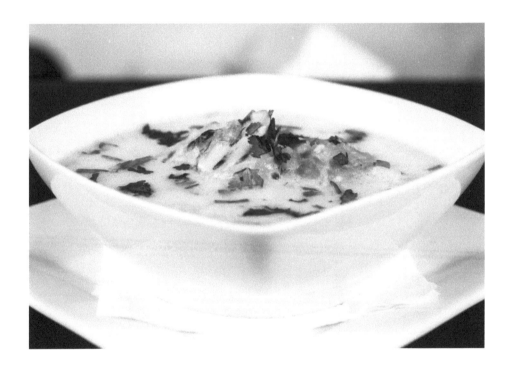

17.   Chorizo Soup

Preparation Time: 10 minutes

Cooking Time: 17 minutes

Servings: 3 servings

Ingredients:

- 8 oz. chorizo, chopped
- 1 teaspoon tomato paste
- 4 oz. scallions, diced
- 1 tablespoon dried cilantro
- ½ teaspoon chili powder
- 1 teaspoon avocado oil
- 2 cups beef broth

Directions:

1. Heat up avocado oil on saute mode for 1 minute.
2. Add chorizo and cook it for 6 minutes, stir it from time to time.
3. Then add scallions, tomato paste, cilantro, and chili powder. Stir well.
4. Add beef broth.
5. Close and seal the lid.
6. Cook the soup on manual mode (high pressure) for 10 minutes. Make a quick pressure release.

Nutrition:

Calories 387 Fat 30.2

Fiber 1.3 Carbs 5.5

Protein 22.3

18.   Red Feta Soup

Preparation Time: 10 minutes

Cooking Time: 25 minutes

Servings: 4 servings

Ingredients:

- 1 cup broccoli, chopped
- 1 teaspoon tomato paste
- ½ cup coconut cream
- 4 cups beef broth
- 1 teaspoon chili flakes
- 6 oz. feta, crumbled

Directions:

1. Put broccoli, tomato paste, coconut cream, and beef broth in the instant pot.
2. Add chili flakes and stir the mixture until it is red.
3. Then close and seal the lid and cook the soup for 8 minutes on manual mode (high pressure).
4. Then make a quick pressure release and open the lid.
5. Add feta cheese and saute the soup on saute mode for 5 minutes more.

Nutrition:

Calories 229 Fat 17.7

Fiber 1.3

Carbs 6.1

Protein 12.3

19. "Ramen" Soup

Preparation Time: 10 minutes **Cooking Time:** 15 minutes

Servings: 2 servings

Ingredients:

- 1 zucchini, trimmed
- 2 cups chicken broth
- 2 eggs, boiled, peeled
- 1 tablespoon coconut aminos
- 5 oz. beef loin, strips
- 1 teaspoon chili flakes
- 1 tablespoon chives, chopped
- ½ teaspoon salt

Directions:

1. Put the beef loin strips in the instant pot.
2. Add chili flakes, salt, and chicken broth.
3. Close and seal the lid. Cook the **Ingredients:** on manual mode (high pressure) for 15 minutes. Make a quick pressure release and open the lid.
4. Then make the s from zucchini with the help of the spiralizer and add them in the soup.
5. Add chives and coconut aminos.
6. Then ladle the soup in the bowls and top with halved eggs.

Nutrition:

Calories 254 Fat 11.8 Fiber 1.1 Carbs 6.2

Protein 30.6

20.   Beef Tagine

Preparation Time: 15 minutes

Cooking Time: 25 minutes

Servings: 6 servings

Ingredients:

- 1-pound beef fillet, chopped

- 1 eggplant, chopped

- 6 oz. scallions, chopped

- 1 teaspoon ground allspices

- 1 teaspoon Erythritol

- 1 teaspoon coconut oil

- 4 cups beef broth

Directions:

1. Put all Ingredients in the instant pot.

2. Close and seal the lid.

3. Cook the meal on manual mode (high pressure) for 25 minutes.

4. Then allow the natural pressure release for 15 minutes.

Nutrition:

Calories 146

Fat 5.3

Fiber 3.5

Carbs 8.8

Protein 16.7

21. Tomatillos Fish Stew

Preparation Time: 15 minutes

Cooking Time: 12 minutes

Servings: 2 servings

Ingredients:

- 2 tomatillos, chopped
- 10 oz. salmon fillet, chopped
- 1 teaspoon ground paprika
- ½ teaspoon ground turmeric
- 1 cup coconut cream
- ½ teaspoon salt

Directions:

1. Put all Ingredients in the instant pot.
2. Close and seal the lid.
3. Cook the fish stew on manual mode (high pressure) for 12 minutes.
4. Then allow the natural pressure release for 10 minutes.

Nutrition:

Calories 479

Fat 37.9

Fiber 3.8

Carbs 9.6

Protein 30.8

22.   Chili Verde Soup

Preparation Time: 10 minutes

Cooking Time: 25 minutes

Servings: 4 servings

Ingredients:

- 2 oz. chili Verde sauce
- ½ cup Cheddar cheese, shredded
- 5 cups chicken broth
- 1-pound chicken breast, skinless, boneless
- 1 tablespoon dried cilantro

Directions:

1. Put chicken breast and chicken broth in the instant pot.
2. Add cilantro, close and seal the lid.
3. Then cook the Ingredients on manual (high pressure) for 15 minutes.
4. Make a quick pressure release and open the li.
5. Shred the chicken breast with the help of the fork.
6. Add dried cilantro and chili Verde sauce in the soup and cook it on saute mode for 10 minutes.
7. Then add dried cilantro and stir well.

Nutrition:

Calories 257 Fat 10.2

Fiber 0.2

Carbs 4

Protein 34.5

23.   Pepper Stuffing Soup

Preparation Time: 10 minutes

Cooking Time: 14 minutes

Servings: 4 servings

Ingredients:

- 1 cup ground beef
- ½ cup cauliflower, shredded
- 1 teaspoon dried oregano
- ½ teaspoon salt
- 1 teaspoon tomato paste
- 1 teaspoon minced garlic
- 4 cups of water
- ¼ cup of coconut milk

Directions:

1. Put all Ingredients in the instant pot bowl and stir well.
2. Then close and seal the lid.
3. Cook the soup on manual mode (high pressure) for 14 minutes.
4. When the time of cooking is finished, make a quick pressure release and open the lid.

Nutrition:

Calories 106 Fat 7.7

Fiber 0.9 Carbs 2.2

Protein 7.3

24.   Steak Soup

Preparation Time: 10 minutes

Cooking Time: 40 minutes

Servings: 5 servings

Ingredients:

- 5 oz. scallions, diced
- 1 tablespoon coconut oil
- 1 oz. daikon, diced
- 1-pound beef round steak, chopped
- 1 teaspoon dried thyme
- 5 cups of water
- ½ teaspoon ground black pepper

Directions:

1. Heat up coconut oil on saute mode for 2 minutes.
2. Add daikon and scallions.
3. After this, stir them well and add chopped beef steak, thyme, and ground black pepper.
4. Saute the Ingredients for 5 minutes more and then add water.
5. Close and seal the lid.
6. Cook the soup on manual mode (high pressure) for 35 minutes. Make a quick pressure release.

Nutrition:

Calories 232 Fat 11 Fiber 0.9

Carbs 2.5 Protein 29.5

25.   Meat Spinach Stew

Preparation Time: 20 minutes

Cooking Time: 30 minutes

Servings: 4 servings

Ingredients:

- 2 cups spinach, chopped
- 1-pound beef sirloin, chopped
- 1 teaspoon allspices
- 3 cups chicken broth
- 1 cup of coconut milk
- 1 teaspoon coconut aminos

Directions:

1. Put all Ingredients in the instant pot.
2. Close and seal the lid.
3. After this, set the manual mode (high pressure) and cook the stew for 30 minutes.
4. When the cooking time is finished, allow the natural pressure release for 10 minutes.
5. Stir the stew gently before serving.

Nutrition:

Calories 383 Fat 22.2

Fiber 1.8

Carbs 5.1

Protein 39.9

26.   Leek Soup

Preparation Time: 10 minutes

Cooking Time: 15 minutes

Servings: 4 servings

Ingredients:

- 7 oz. leek, chopped
- 2 oz. Monterey Jack cheese, shredded
- 1 teaspoon Italian seasonings
- ½ teaspoon salt
- 4 tablespoons butter
- 2 cups chicken broth

Directions:

1. Heat up butter in the instant pot for 4 minutes.
2. Then add chopped leek, salt, and Italian seasonings.
3. Cook the leek on saute mode for 5 minutes. Stir the vegetables from time to time.
4. After this, add chicken broth and close the lid.
5. Cook the soup on saute mode for 10 minutes.
6. Then add shredded cheese and stir it till the cheese is melted.
7. The soup is cooked.

Nutrition:

Calories 208 Fat 17

Fiber 0.9

Carbs 7.7

Protein 6.8

CHAPTER 5:

Poultry

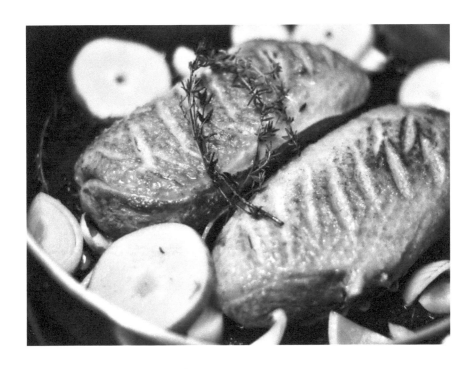

27. Boozy Glazed Chicken

Preparation Time: 40 minutes

Cooking Time: 1 hour + marinating time

Servings: 4

Ingredients:

- 2 pounds chicken drumettes
- 2 tablespoons ghee, at room temperature
- Sea salt and ground black pepper, to taste
- 1 teaspoon Mediterranean seasoning mix
- 2 vine-ripened tomatoes, pureed
- 3/4 cup rum
- 3 tablespoons coconut aminos
- A few drops of liquid Stevia
- 1 teaspoon chile peppers, minced
- 1 tablespoon minced fresh ginger
- 1 teaspoon ground cardamom
- 2 tablespoons fresh lemon juice, plus wedges for serving

Directions:

1. Toss the chicken with the melted ghee, salt, black pepper, and Mediterranean seasoning mix until well coated on all sides.

2. In another bowl, thoroughly combine the pureed tomato puree, rum, coconut aminos, Stevia, chile peppers, ginger, cardamom, and lemon juice.

3. Pour the tomato mixture over the chicken drumettes; let it marinate for 2 hours. Bake in the preheated oven at 410 degrees F for about 45 minutes.

4. Add in the reserved marinade and place under the preheated broiler for 10 minutes.

Nutrition:

307 Calories

12.1g Fat

2.7g Carbs

33.6g Protein

1.5g Fiber

28.   Festive Turkey Rouladen

Preparation Time: 15 minutes **Cooking Time:** 30 minutes

Servings: 5

Ingredients:

- 2 pounds turkey fillet, marinated and cut into 10 pieces
- 10 strips prosciutto
- 1/2 teaspoon chili powder
- 1 teaspoon marjoram
- 1 sprig rosemary, finely chopped
- 2 tablespoons dry white wine
- 1 teaspoon garlic, finely minced
- 1 ½ tablespoons butter, room temperature
- 1 tablespoon Dijon mustard
- Sea salt and freshly ground black pepper, to your liking

Directions:

1. Start by preheating your oven to 430 degrees F.
2. Pat the turkey dry and cook in hot butter for about 3 minutes per side. Add in the mustard, chili powder, marjoram, rosemary, wine, and garlic.
3. Continue to cook for 2 minutes more. Wrap each turkey piece into one prosciutto strip and secure with toothpicks.
4. Roast in the preheated oven for about 30 minutes.

Nutrition:

286 Calories 9.7g Fat 6.9g Carbs

39.9g Protein 0.3g Fiber

29. Pan-Fried Chorizo Sausage

Preparation Time: 10 minutes **Cooking Time:** 20 minutes

Servings: 4

Ingredients:

- 16 ounces smoked turkey chorizo
- 1 ½ cups Asiago cheese, grated
- 1 teaspoon oregano
- 1 teaspoon basil
- 1 cup tomato puree
- 4 scallion stalks, chopped
- 1 teaspoon garlic paste
- Sea salt and ground black pepper, to taste
- 1 tablespoon dry sherry
- 1 tablespoon extra-virgin olive oil
- 2 tablespoons fresh coriander, roughly chopped

Directions:

1. Heat the oil in a frying pan over moderately high heat. Now, brown the turkey chorizo, crumbling with a fork for about 5 minutes.
2. Add in the other Ingredients, except for cheese; continue to cook for 10 minutes more or until cooked through.

Nutrition:

330 Calories 17.2g Fat 4.5g Carbs

34.4g Protein 1.6g Fiber

30. Chinese Bok Choy and Turkey Soup

Preparation Time: 15 minutes

Cooking Time: 40 minutes

Servings: 8

Ingredients:

- 1/2 pound baby Bok choy, sliced into quarters lengthwise
- 2 pounds turkey carcass
- 1 tablespoon olive oil
- 1/2 cup leeks, chopped
- 1 celery rib, chopped
- 2 carrots, sliced
- 6 cups turkey stock
- Himalayan salt and black pepper, to taste

Directions:

1. In a heavy-bottomed pot, heat the olive oil until sizzling. Once hot, sauté the celery, carrots, leek and Bok choy for about 6 minutes.
2. Add the salt, pepper, turkey, and stock; bring to a boil.
3. Turn the heat to simmer. Continue to cook, partially covered, for about 35 minutes.

Nutrition:

211 Calories 11.8g Fat

3.1g Carbs 23.7g Protein

0.9g Fiber

CHAPTER 6:

Beef Recipes

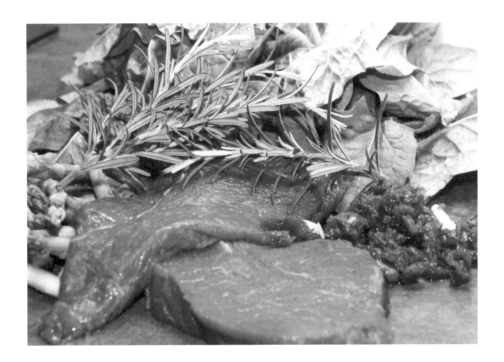

31.   Beef and Sausage Medley

Preparation Time: 10 minutes

Cooking Time: 27 minutes

Servings: 8

Ingredients:

- 1 teaspoon butter
- 2 beef sausages, casing removed and sliced
- 2 pounds (907 g) beef steak, cubed
- 1 yellow onion, sliced
- 2 fresh ripe tomatoes, puréed
- 1 jalapeño pepper, chopped
- 1 red bell pepper, chopped
- 1½ cups roasted vegetable broth
- 2 cloves garlic, minced
- 1 teaspoon Old Bay seasoning
- 2 bay leaves
- 1 sprig thyme
- 1 sprig rosemary
- ½ teaspoon paprika
- Sea salt and ground black pepper, to taste

Directions:

1. Press the Sauté button to heat up the Instant Pot. Melt the butter and cook the sausage and steak for 4 minutes, stirring periodically. Set aside.

2. Add the onion and sauté for 3 minutes or until softened and translucent. Add the remaining ingredients, including reserved beef and sausage.

3. Secure the lid. Choose Manual mode and set time for 20 minutes on High Pressure.

4. Once cooking is complete, use a quick pressure release. Carefully remove the lid.

5. Serve immediately.

Nutrition:

Calories: 319

Fat: 14.0g

Protein: 42.8g

Carbs: 6.3g

Net carbs: 1.8g

Fiber: 4.5g

32.   Beef Back Ribs with Barbecue Glaze

Preparation Time: 10 minutes

Cooking Time: 35 minutes

Servings: 4

Ingredients:

- ½ cup water
- 1 (3-pound / 1.4-kg) rack beef back ribs, prepared with rub of choice
- ¼ cup unsweetened tomato purée
- ¼ teaspoon Worcestershire sauce
- ¼ teaspoon garlic powder
- 2 teaspoons apple cider vinegar
- ¼ teaspoon liquid smoke
- ¼ teaspoon smoked paprika
- 3 tablespoons Swerve
- Dash of cayenne pepper

Directions:

1. Pour the water in the pot and place the trivet inside.
2. Arrange the ribs on top of the trivet.
3. Close the lid. Select Manual mode and set cooking time for 25 minutes on High Pressure.
4. Meanwhile, prepare the glaze by whisking together the tomato purée, Worcestershire sauce, garlic powder, vinegar, liquid smoke, paprika, Swerve, and cayenne in a medium bowl. Heat the broiler.

5. When timer beeps, quick release the pressure. Open the lid. Remove the ribs and place on a baking sheet.

6. Brush a layer of glaze on the ribs. Put under the broiler for 5 minutes.

7. Remove from the broiler and brush with glaze again. Put back under the broiler for 5 more minutes, or until the tops are sticky.

8. Serve immediately.

Nutrition:

Calories: 758

Fat: 26.8g

Protein: 33.7g

Carbs: 0.9g

Net carbs: 0.7g

Fiber: 0.2g

33. Beef Big Mac Salad

Preparation Time: 10 minutes

Cooking Time: 9 minutes

Servings: 2

Ingredients:

- 5 ounces (142 g) ground beef
- 1 teaspoon ground black pepper
- 1 tablespoon sesame oil
- 1 cup lettuce, chopped
- ¼ cup Monterey Jack cheese, shredded
- 2 ounces (57 g) dill pickles, sliced
- 1 ounce (28 g) scallions, chopped
- 1 tablespoon heavy cream

Directions:

1. In a mixing bowl, combine the ground beef and ground black pepper. Shape the mixture into mini burgers.
2. Pour the sesame oil in the Instant Pot and heat for 3 minutes on Sauté mode.
3. Place the mini hamburgers in the hot oil and cook for 3 minutes on each side.
4. Meanwhile, in a salad bowl, mix the chopped lettuce, shredded cheese, dill pickles, scallions, and heavy cream. Toss to mix well.
5. Top the salad with cooked mini burgers. Serve immediately.

Nutrition:

Calories: 284

Fat: 18.5g

Protein: 25.7g

Carbs: 3.5g

Net carbs: 2.3g

Fiber: 1.2g

CHAPTER 7:

Pork Recipes

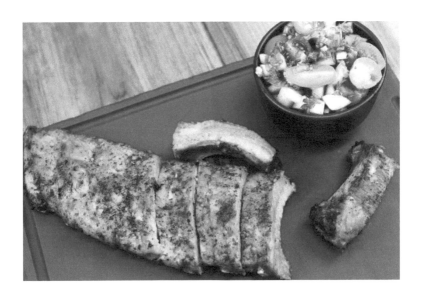

34.   Classic Sausage and Peppers

Preparation Time: 10 Minutes

Cooking Time: 35 Minutes

Servings: 6

Ingredients:

- 1½ pounds sweet Italian sausages (or hot if you prefer)
- 2 tablespoons good-quality olive oil
- 1 red bell pepper, cut into thin strips
- 1 yellow bell pepper, cut into thin strips
- 1 orange bell pepper, cut into thin strips
- 1 red onion, thinly sliced
- 1 tablespoon minced garlic
- ½ cup white wine
- Sea salt, for seasoning
- Freshly ground black pepper, for seasoning

Directions:

1. Cook the sausage. Preheat a grill to medium-high and grill the sausages, turning them several times, until they're cooked through, about 12 minutes in total. Let the sausages rest for 15 minutes and then cut them into 2-inch pieces.

2. Sauté the vegetables. In a large skillet over medium-high heat, warm the olive oil. Add the red, yellow, and orange bell peppers, and the red onion and garlic and sauté until they're tender, about 10 minutes.

3. Finish the dish. Add the sausage to the skillet along with the white wine and sauté for 10 minutes.

4. Serve. Divide the mixture between four plates, season it with salt and pepper, and serve.

Nutrition:

Calories: 450

Total fat: 40g

Total carbs: 5g

Fiber: 1g;

Net carbs: 4g

Sodium: 554mg

Protein: 17g

35. Lemon-Infused Pork Rib Roast

Preparation Time: 10 Minutes

Cooking Time: 1 Hour

Servings: 6

Ingredients:

- ¼ cup good-quality olive oil
- Zest and juice of 1 lemon
- Zest and juice of 1 orange
- 4 rosemary sprigs, lightly crushed
- 4 thyme sprigs, lightly crushed
- 1 (4-bone) pork rib roast, about 2½ pounds
- 6 garlic cloves, peeled
- Sea salt, for seasoning
- Freshly ground black pepper, for seasoning

Directions:

1. Make the marinade. In a large bowl, combine the olive oil, lemon zest, lemon juice, orange zest, orange juice, rosemary sprigs, and thyme sprigs.

2. Marinate the roast. Use a small knife to make six 1-inch-deep slits in the fatty side of the roast. Stuff the garlic cloves in the slits. Put the roast in the bowl with the marinade and turn it to coat it well with the marinade. Cover the bowl and refrigerate it overnight, turning the roast in the marinade several times.

3. Preheat the oven. Set the oven temperature to 350°F.

4. Roast the pork. Remove the pork from the marinade and season it with salt and pepper, then put it in a baking dish and let it come to room temperature. Roast the pork until it's cooked through (145°F to 160°F internal temperature), about 1 hour. Throw out any leftover marinade.

5. Serve. Let the pork rest for 10 minutes, then cut it into slices and arrange the slices on a platter. Serve it warm.

Nutrition:

Calories: 403

Total fat: 30g

Total carbs: 1g

Fiber: 0g;

Net carbs: 1g

Sodium: 113mg

Protein: 30g

CHAPTER 8:

Lamb Recipes

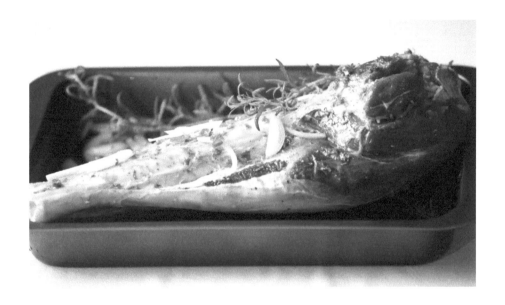

36. Lamb in Almond Sauce

Preparation Time: 10 minutes

Cooking Time: 30 minutes

Servings: 6

Ingredients:

- 14 oz. lamb fillet, cubed
- 1 cup organic almond milk
- 1 teaspoon almond flour
- 1 teaspoon ground nutmeg
- ½ teaspoon ground cardamom
- 1 tablespoon olive oil
- 1 tablespoon lemon juice
- 1 tablespoon butter
- ½ teaspoon minced garlic

Directions:

1. Preheat the olive oil in the saucepan.
2. Meanwhile, mix lamb, ground nutmeg, ground cardamom, and minced garlic.
3. Put the lamb in the hot olive oil. Roast the meat for 2 minutes per side.
4. Then add butter, lemon juice, and almond milk. Carefully mix the mixture.
5. Cook the meal for 15 minutes on medium heat.
6. Then add almond flour, stir well and simmer the meal for 10 minutes more.

Nutrition:

Calories 258

Fat 19

Fiber 1.1

Carbs 2.7

Protein 19.7

37. Sweet Leg of Lamb

Preparation Time: 10 minutes

Cooking Time: 45 minutes

Servings: 6

Ingredients:

- 2 pounds lamb leg
- 1 tablespoon Erythritol
- 3 tablespoons coconut milk
- 1 teaspoon chili flakes
- 1 teaspoon ground turmeric
- 1 teaspoon cayenne pepper
- 3 tablespoons coconut oil

Directions:

1. In the shallow bowl, mix cayenne pepper, ground turmeric, chili flakes, and Erythritol.
2. Rub the lamb leg with spices.
3. Melt the coconut oil in the saucepan.
4. Add lamb leg and roast it for 10 minutes per side on low heat.
5. After this, add coconut milk and cook the meal for 30 minutes on low heat. Flip the meat on another side from time to time.

Nutrition:

Calories 350 Fat 18.8 Fiber 0.3

Carbs 0.8 Protein 42.8

38.   Coconut Lamb Shoulder

Preparation Time: 10 minutes

Cooking Time: 75 minutes

Servings: 5

Ingredients:

- 2-pound lamb shoulder
- 1 teaspoon ground cumin
- 2 tablespoons butter
- ¼ cup of coconut milk
- 1 teaspoon coconut shred
- ½ cup kale, chopped

Directions:

1. Put all ingredients in the saucepan and mix well.
2. Close the lid and cook the meal on low heat for 75 minutes.

Nutrition:

Calories 414

Fat 21.2

Fiber 0.5

Carbs 1.7

Protein 51.5

CHAPTER 9:

Seafood

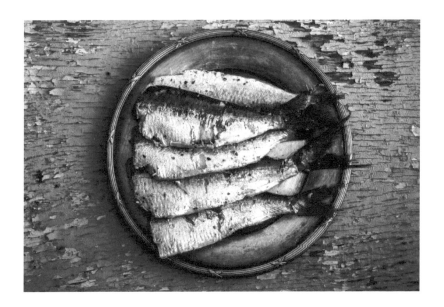

39. Tuna Salad Pickle Boats

Preparation Time: 10 minutes

Cooking Time: 0 minutes;

Servings: 2

Ingredients

- 4 dill pickles
- 4 oz. of tuna, packed in water, drained
- ¼ of lime, juiced
- 4 tbsp. mayonnaise
- Seasoning:
- ¼ tsp salt
- 1/8 tsp ground black pepper
- ¼ tsp paprika
- 1 tbsp. mustard paste

Directions:

1. Prepare tuna salad and for this, take a medium bowl, place tuna in it, add lime juice, mayonnaise, salt, black pepper, paprika, and mustard and stir until mixed.
2. Cut each pickle into half lengthwise, scoop out seeds, and then fill with tuna salad.
3. Serve.

Nutrition: 308.5 Calories; 23.7 g Fats; 17 g Protein; 3.8 g Net Carb; 3.1 g Fiber;

40.   Shrimp Deviled Eggs

Preparation Time: 5 minutes

Cooking Time: 0 minutes;

Servings: 2

Ingredients

- 2 eggs, boiled
- 2 oz. shrimps, cooked, chopped
- ½ tsp tabasco sauce
- ½ tsp mustard paste
- 2 tbsp. mayonnaise
- Seasoning:
- 1/8 tsp salt
- 1/8 tsp ground black pepper

Directions:

1. Peel the boiled eggs, then slice in half lengthwise and transfer egg yolks to a medium bowl by using a spoon.
2. Mash the egg yolk, add remaining ingredients and stir until well combined.
3. Spoon the egg yolk mixture into egg whites, and then serve.

Nutrition: 210 Calories; 16.4 g Fats; 14 g Protein; 1 g Net Carb; 0.1 g Fiber;

41.   Herb Crusted Tilapia

Preparation Time: 5 minutes

Cooking Time: 10 minutes;

Servings: 2

Ingredients

- 2 fillets of tilapia
- ½ tsp garlic powder
- ½ tsp Italian seasoning
- ½ tsp dried parsley
- 1/3 tsp salt
- Seasoning:
- 2 tbsp. melted butter, unsalted
- 1 tbsp. avocado oil

Directions:

1. Turn on the broiler and then let it preheat.
2. Meanwhile, take a small bowl, place melted butter in it, stir in oil and garlic powder until mixed, and then brush this mixture over tilapia fillets.
3. Stir together remaining spices and then sprinkle them generously on tilapia until well coated.
4. Place seasoned tilapia in a baking pan, place the pan under the broiler and then bake for 10 minutes until tender and golden, brushing with garlic-butter every 2 minutes.

5. Serve.

Nutrition: 520 Calories; 35 g Fats; 36.2 g Protein; 13.6 g Net Carb; 0.6 g Fiber;

CHAPTER 10:

Vegetables

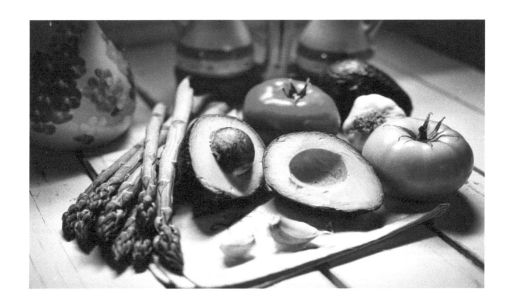

42. Sautéed Crispy Zucchini

Preparation Time: 15 minutes

Cooking Time: 10 minutes

Servings: 4

Ingredients:

- 2 tablespoons butter
- 4 zucchini, cut into ¼-inch-thick rounds
- ½ cup freshly grated Parmesan cheese
- Freshly ground black pepper

Directions:

1. Place a large skillet over medium-high heat and melt the butter.
2. Add the zucchini and sauté until tender and lightly browned, about 5 minutes.
3. Spread the zucchini evenly in the skillet and sprinkle the Parmesan cheese over the vegetables.
4. Cook without stirring until the Parmesan cheese is melted and crispy where it touches the skillet, about 5 minutes
5. Serve.

Nutrition:

Calories: 94 Fat: 8g

Protein: 4g Carbs: 1g

Fiber: 0g Net Carbs: 1g

Fat 76

Protein 20

Carbs 4

43. Mushrooms with Camembert

Preparation Time: 5 minutes

Cooking Time: 15 minutes

Servings: 4

Ingredients:

- 2 tablespoons butter
- 2 teaspoons minced garlic
- 1 pound button mushrooms, halved
- 4 ounces Camembert cheese, diced
- Freshly ground black pepper

Directions:

1. Place a large skillet over medium-high heat and melt the butter.
2. Sauté the garlic until translucent, about 3 minutes.
3. Sauté the mushrooms until tender, about 10 minutes.
4. Stir in the cheese and sauté until melted, about 2 minutes.
5. Season with pepper and serve.

Nutrition:

Calories: 161 Fat: 13g

Protein: 9g Carbs: 4g

Fiber: 1g

Net Carbs: 3g

Fat 70

Protein 21

Carbs 9

CHAPTER 11:

Snacks

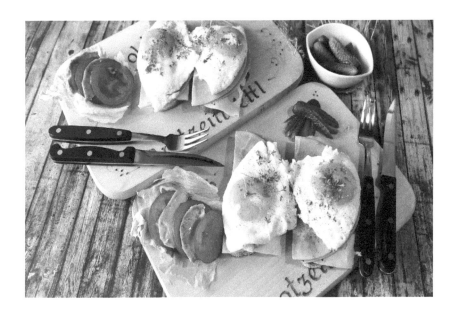

44. Pumpkin Muffins.

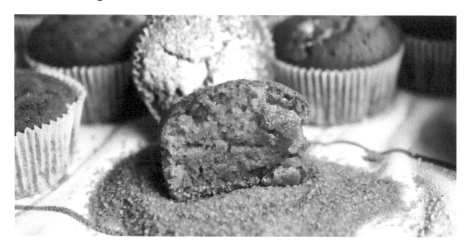

Preparation Time: 10 minutes

Cooking Time: 15 minutes

Servings: 18

Ingredients:

- ¼ cup sunflower seed butter
- ¾ cup pumpkin puree 2 tablespoons flaxseed meal ¼ cup coconut flour
- ½ cup erythritol ½ teaspoon nutmeg, ground
- 1 teaspoon cinnamon, ground ½ teaspoon baking soda 1 egg ½ teaspoon baking powder
- A pinch of salt

Directions:

1. In a bowl, mix butter with pumpkin puree and egg and blend well.

2. Add flaxseed meal, coconut flour, erythritol, baking soda, baking powder, nutmeg, cinnamon and a pinch of salt and stir well.

3. Spoon this into a greased muffin pan, introduce in the oven at 350 degrees F and bake for 15 minutes.

4. Leave muffins to cool down and serve them as a snack.

5. Enjoy!

Nutrition:

Calories: 65 kcal

Protein: 2.82 g

Fat: 5.42 g

Carbohydrates: 2.27 g

Sodium: 57 mg

45. Creamy Mango and Mint Dip

Preparation Time: 10 minutes

Cooking Time: 15 minutes

Servings 4

Ingredients:

- Medium green chili, chopped – 1
- Medium white onion, peeled and chopped – 1
- Grated ginger – 1 tablespoon
- Minced garlic – 1 teaspoon
- Salt – 1/8 teaspoon
- Ground black pepper – 1/8 teaspoon
- Cumin powder – 1 teaspoon
- Mango powder – 1 teaspoon
- Mint leaves – 2 cups
- Coriander leaves – 1 cup
- Cashew yogurt – 4 tablespoons

Directions:

1. Place all the ingredients for the dip in a blender and pulse for 1 to 2 minutes or until smooth.
2. Tip the dip into small cups and serve straightaway.

Nutrition: calories: 100, fat: 2, fiber: 3, carbs: 7, protein: 5

46. Hot Red Chili and Garlic Chutney

Preparation Time: 25 minutes

Cooking Time: 15 minutes

Servings 1

Ingredients:

- Red chilies, dried – 14
- Minced garlic – 5 teaspoons
- Salt – 1/8 teaspoon
- Water – 1 and ¼ cups

Directions:

1. Place chilies in a bowl, pour in water and let rest for 20 minutes.
2. Then drain red chilies, chop them and add to a blender.
3. Add remaining ingredients into the blender and pulse for 1 to 2 minutes until smooth.
4. Tip the sauce into a bowl and serve straight away.

Nutrition: calories: 100, fat: 1, fiber: 2, carbs: 6, protein: 7

47. Red Chilies and Onion Chutney

Preparation Time: 15 minutes

Cooking Time: 15 minutes

Servings 2

Ingredients:

- Medium white onion, peeled and chopped – 1

- Minced garlic – 1 teaspoon

- Red chilies, chopped – 2

- Salt – ¼ teaspoon

- Sweet paprika – 1 teaspoon

- Avocado oil – 2 teaspoons

- Water – ¼ cup

Directions:

1. Place a medium skillet pan over medium-high heat, add oil and when hot, add onion, garlic, and chilies.

2. Cook onions for 5 minutes or until softened, then season with salt and paprika and pour in water.

3. Stir well and cook for 5 minutes.

4. Then spoon the chutney into a bowl and serve.

Nutrition: calories: 121, fat: 2, fiber: 6, carbs: 9, protein: 5

48.   Fast Guacamole

Preparation Time: 10 minutes

Cooking Time: 15 minutes

Servings 12

Ingredients:

- Medium avocados, peeled, pitted and cubed – 3
- Medium tomato, cubed – 1
- Chopped cilantro – ¼ cup
- Medium red onion, peeled and chopped – 1
- Salt – ½ teaspoon
- Ground white pepper – ¼ teaspoon
- Lime juice – 3 tablespoons

Directions:

1. Place all the ingredients for the salad in a medium bowl and stir until combined.
2. Serve guacamole straightaway as an appetizer.

Nutrition: calories: 87, fat: 4, fiber: 4, carbs: 8, protein: 2

.

CHAPTER 12:

Desserts

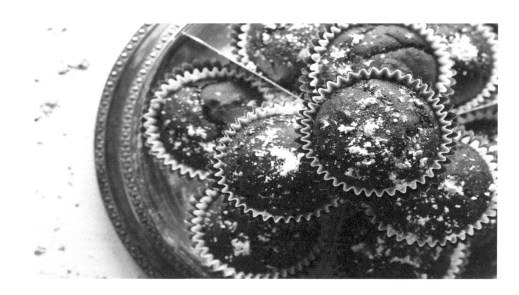

49. Strawberry Angel Food Dessert

Difficulty: Novice level

Preparation Time: 15 minutes

Cooking Time: 0 minutes

Servings: 18

Size/ Portion: 1 cup

Ingredients

- 1 angel cake (10 inches)
- 2 packages of softened cream cheese
- 1 cup of white sugar
- 1 container (8 oz.) of frozen fluff, thawed
- 1 liter of fresh strawberries, sliced
- 1 jar of strawberry icing

Direction

1. Crumble the cake in a 9 x 13-inch dish.
2. Beat the cream cheese and sugar in a medium bowl until the mixture is light and fluffy. Stir in the whipped topping. Crush the cake with your hands, and spread the cream cheese mixture over the cake.
3. Combine the strawberries and the frosting in a bowl until the strawberries are well covered. Spread over the layer of cream cheese. Cool until ready to serve.

Nutrition:

261 calories 11g fat 3.2g protein

50. Rhubarb Strawberry Crunch

Preparation Time: 15 minutes **Cooking Time:** 45 minutes

Servings: 18

Size/ Portion: 1 cup

Ingredients

- 1 cup of white sugar

- 3 tablespoons all-purpose flour

- 3 cups of fresh strawberries, sliced

- 3 cups of rhubarb, cut into cubes

- 1 1/2 cup flour

- 1 cup packed brown sugar

- 1 cup butter

- 1 cup oatmeal

Direction

1. Preheat the oven to 190 ° C.

2. Combine white sugar, 3 tablespoons flour, strawberries and rhubarb in a large bowl. Place the mixture in a 9 x 13-inch baking dish.

3. Mix 1 1/2 cups of flour, brown sugar, butter, and oats until a crumbly texture is obtained. You may want to use a blender for this. Crumble the mixture of rhubarb and strawberry.Bake for 45 minutes.

Nutrition:

253 calories 10.8g fat 2.3g protein

51.   Chocolate Chip Banana Dessert

Preparation Time: 20 minutes

Cooking Time: 20 minutes

Servings: 24

Size/ Portion:

Ingredients

- 2/3 cup white sugar

- 3/4 cup butter

- 2/3 cup brown sugar

- 1 egg, beaten slightly

- 1 teaspoon vanilla extract

- 1 cup of banana puree

- 1 3/4 cup flour

- 2 teaspoons baking powder

- 1/2 teaspoon of salt

- 1 cup of semi-sweet chocolate chips

Direction:

1. Ready the oven to 175 ° C Grease and bake a 10 x 15-inch baking pan.

2. Beat the butter, white sugar, and brown sugar in a large bowl until light. Beat the egg and vanilla. Fold in the banana puree: mix baking powder, flour, and salt in another bowl. Mix flour

mixture into the butter mixture. Stir in the chocolate chips. Spread in pan.

3. Bake for 20 minutes. Cool before cutting into squares.

Nutrition:

174 calories

8.2g fat

1.7g protein

52.   Apple Pie Filling

Preparation Time: 20 minutes

Cooking Time: 12 minutes

Servings: 40

Size/ Portion: 1 cup

Ingredients

- 18 cups chopped apples
- 3 tablespoons lemon juice
- 10 cups of water
- 4 1/2 cups of white sugar
- 1 cup corn flour
- 2 teaspoons of ground cinnamon
- 1 teaspoon of salt
- 1/4 teaspoon ground nutmeg

Direction

1. Mix apples with lemon juice in a large bowl and set aside. Pour the water in a Dutch oven over medium heat. Combine sugar, corn flour, cinnamon, salt, and nutmeg in a bowl. Add to water, mix well, and bring to a boil. Cook for 2 minutes with continuous stirring.

2. Boil apples again. Reduce the heat, cover, and simmer for 8 minutes. Allow cooling for 30 minutes.

3. Pour into five freezer containers and leave 1/2 inch of free space. Cool to room temperature.

4. Seal and freeze

Nutrition:

129 calories

0.1g fat

0.2g protein

Conclusion

Thanks for downloading this book. In this book, you were provided a variety of keto-friendly recipes. From cooking keto-friendly breakfast, lunch, and dinner, to fun different takes on snacking and yummy desserts, this book offers all the variety for a healthy, well-rounded diet plan. Be sure to keep the diet plan and the keto-shopping list nearby to make things easier. The recipes in this book are not just simple to understand but will help you whip up delicious and nutritious meals in no time.

With Ketogenic diet, you have to avoid or limit your consumption of carbs to less than 5% of your daily dietary intake. Secondly, you need to avoid unhealthy carbs such as tubers, starches, sugar, and other foods.

Once you have all of the chief spices and other fixings stocked in your keto kitchen, the following week's shopping list will be much simpler. As a quick reminder, keep these simple tips in mind as you go through your ketogenic journey:

Drink plenty of water daily and limit the intake of sugar-sweetened beverages.

It is essential to attempt to use only half of your typical serving of salad dressing or butter.

Use only fat-free or low-fat condiments.

Add a serving of vegetables to your dinner and lunch menus.

Add a serving of fruit as a snack or enjoy with your meal. The skin also contains additional nutrients. Dried and canned fruits are quick and easy to use. However, make sure they don't have added sugar.

Read the food labels and make choices that keep you in line with ketosis.

A snack has some frozen yogurt (fat-free or low-fat), nuts or unsalted pretzels, raw veggies, and unsalted-plain popcorn.

Prepare cut veggies such as bell pepper strips, mixed greens, and carrots. Store them in small baggies for a quick on-the-go healthy choice.

One of the easiest ways to stay on your plan is to remove the temptations. Remove the chocolate, candy, bread, pasta, rice, and sugary sodas you have supplied in your kitchen. If you live alone, this is an easy task. It is a bit more challenging if you have a family. The diet will also be useful for them if you plan your meals using the recipes included in this book.

If you cheat, that has to count also. It will be a reminder of your indulgence, but it will help keep you in line. Others may believe you are obsessed with the plan, but it is your health and wellbeing that you are improving.

When you go shopping for your ketogenic essentials be sure you take your new skills, a grocery list, and search the labels. Almost every food item in today's grocery store has a nutrition label. Be sure you read each ingredient to discover any hiding carbs to keep your ketosis in line. You will be glad you took the extra time.

CPSIA information can be obtained
at www.ICGtesting.com
Printed in the USA
LVHW071043130221
679242LV00001B/3